Cold and Flu Natural Home Remedies

Dr. Harry Rusden

Copyright © 2024 Dr. Harry Rusden
Alright reserved

Table of Contents

1. **Introduction**
   - Understanding the Common Cold and Influenza
   - Importance of Natural Home Remedies

2. **Preventive Measures**
   - Boosting Immunity through Diet and Lifestyle Changes
   - Hygiene Practices to Prevent Cold and Flu

3. **Herbal Remedies**
   - Echinacea: Benefits and Usage
   - Elderberry Syrup: An Immune-Boosting Elixir
   - Garlic: Nature's Antibiotic
   - Ginger: Soothing and Anti-inflammatory Properties

4. **Vitamins and Supplements**
   - Vitamin C: Immune Support and Symptom Relief
   - Zinc: Shortening Cold Duration and Reducing Severity
   - Vitamin D: Enhancing Immune Function

5. **Hydration and Warmth**
   - Importance of Adequate Hydration
   - Hot Liquids: Herbal Teas, Broths, and Soups

6. Steam Therapy and Inhalation
   - Steam Inhalation with Essential Oils
   - Nasal Irrigation with Saline Solution

7. Rest and Sleep
   - The Healing Power of Rest
   - Creating a Comfortable Sleeping Environment

8. Humidification
   - Using Humidifiers to Relieve Congestion
   - Natural Humidification Methods

9. Nutrition and Diet
   - Foods to Eat During Cold and Flu
   - Foods to Avoid

10. Alternative Therapies
   - Acupuncture: Balancing Energy Flow
   - Homeopathy: Individualized Treatment for Symptoms

11. Exercise and Movement
   - Gentle Exercise for Symptom Relief
   - Yoga and Stretching for Relaxation

12. Home Remedies for Children

- Safe and Effective Remedies for Kids
  - Dosage and Precautions

13. **When to Seek Medical Attention**
    - Signs of Complications
    - Consulting a Healthcare Professional

14. **Conclusion**
    - Recap of Key Points
    - Empowering Self-Care Practices for Cold and Flu

Introduction

The common cold and influenza, often referred to as the flu, are widespread respiratory illnesses caused by viruses. These ailments can disrupt daily life, causing symptoms such as congestion, coughing, sore throat, fatigue, and fever. While over-the-counter medications are commonly used for relief, natural home remedies offer effective alternatives with fewer side effects.

Understanding the principles behind natural remedies for cold and flu empowers individuals to take proactive steps in managing their health. From boosting immunity through diet and lifestyle adjustments to harnessing the healing properties of herbs and supplements, this guide provides comprehensive insights into holistic approaches for prevention and symptom relief.

By incorporating these natural remedies into daily routines, individuals can minimize the impact of cold and flu, promoting overall well-being and resilience against seasonal illnesses. This guide serves as a valuable resource for those seeking safe, accessible, and effective strategies to support their immune system and alleviate symptoms naturally.

Understanding the Common Cold and Influenza

The common cold and influenza are respiratory illnesses caused by viruses, but they differ in severity, duration, and specific symptoms.

1. **Common Cold**:
    - Typically caused by rhinoviruses, but can also be triggered by other viruses.
    - Symptoms include a runny or stuffy nose, sneezing, sore throat, cough, mild fatigue, and occasionally a low-grade fever.
    - Cold symptoms usually develop gradually and are milder compared to the flu.
    - Recovery time varies but generally lasts from a few days to a week.

2. **Influenza (Flu)**:
    - Caused by influenza viruses (types A, B, and rarely C).
    - Symptoms are more severe and sudden onset compared to the common cold and may include high fever, body aches, chills, fatigue, headache, and a dry cough.
    - Complications such as pneumonia, sinus infections, and worsening of chronic medical conditions are more common with the flu.

- Recovery time can range from a week to several weeks, depending on the individual's health and the severity of the illness.

Understanding the differences between these respiratory illnesses is crucial for proper management and treatment. While both cold and flu are contagious and spread through respiratory droplets, preventive measures and natural remedies can help reduce the risk of infection and alleviate symptoms effectively.

Importance of Natural Home Remedies

1. **Minimal Side Effects**: Natural remedies often have fewer side effects compared to over-the-counter medications, making them safer for long-term use and suitable for individuals with sensitivities or allergies.

2. **Supports Immune System**: Many natural remedies work by supporting the body's immune response, helping to strengthen the immune system's ability to fight off viruses and infections.

3. **Accessible and Affordable**: Most natural remedies can be easily found in households or

purchased at affordable prices from local stores or markets, making them accessible to a wide range of individuals.

4. **Holistic Approach**: Natural remedies often take a holistic approach to health, addressing not only symptoms but also underlying imbalances in the body, promoting overall well-being.

5. **Customizable**: Natural remedies can be tailored to individual preferences and needs, allowing for personalized treatment plans that cater to specific symptoms and health conditions.

6. **Reduced Dependency on Medications**: By incorporating natural remedies into daily routines, individuals may reduce their reliance on medications, leading to a more sustainable approach to managing health.

7. **Promotes Self-Care**: Using natural remedies encourages individuals to take an active role in their health and well-being, fostering a sense of empowerment and self-sufficiency.

8. **Environmentally Friendly**: Many natural remedies are derived from plants and herbs, making them environmentally friendly alternatives

to synthetic medications that may have a larger ecological footprint.

Overall, natural home remedies offer a gentle yet effective approach to managing common ailments such as colds and flu, promoting health and wellness in a sustainable and accessible manner.

Chapter 1

Preventive Measures

1. **Boosting Immunity through Diet and Nutrition**:
   - Incorporate immune-boosting foods rich in vitamins (e.g., fruits, vegetables), minerals (e.g., zinc, selenium), and antioxidants (e.g., berries, green tea).
   - Maintain a balanced diet to support overall health and immune function.

2. **Hygiene Practices**:
   - Wash hands frequently with soap and water for at least 20 seconds, especially before eating, after using the restroom, and after coughing or sneezing.
   - Use hand sanitizer with at least 60% alcohol when handwashing is not possible.
   - Avoid touching the face, especially the eyes, nose, and mouth, to prevent the spread of viruses.

3. **Proper Respiratory Etiquette**:
   - Cover mouth and nose with a tissue or elbow when coughing or sneezing.
   - Dispose of used tissues properly and wash hands immediately afterward.

- Avoid close contact with individuals who are sick, and stay home if experiencing symptoms.

4. **Adequate Rest and Sleep**:
   - Prioritize regular sleep schedules and aim for 7-9 hours of quality sleep per night to support immune function and overall health.

5. **Stress Management**:
   - Practice stress-reducing techniques such as meditation, deep breathing exercises, yoga, or hobbies to reduce the impact of stress on immune function.

6. **Regular Exercise**:
   - Engage in moderate physical activity most days of the week to enhance immune function and overall well-being.
   - Maintain social distancing and follow safety guidelines when exercising in public spaces.

7. **Stay Hydrated**:
   - Drink plenty of fluids, such as water, herbal teas, and broths, to stay hydrated and support mucous membrane health.

8. **Environmental Considerations**:
   - Keep indoor environments well-ventilated to reduce the concentration of airborne viruses.
   - Clean and disinfect frequently-touched surfaces regularly, including doorknobs, light switches, and electronic devices.

By implementing these preventive measures, individuals can reduce their risk of contracting and spreading colds and flu viruses, promoting a healthier environment for themselves and others.

Boosting Immunity through Diet and Lifestyle Changes

1. **Nutrient-Rich Diet**:
   - Incorporate a variety of fruits, vegetables, whole grains, lean proteins, and healthy fats into daily meals.
   - Focus on foods rich in immune-boosting vitamins and minerals, including vitamin C (citrus fruits, bell peppers), vitamin D (fatty fish, fortified foods), zinc (lean meats, nuts, seeds), and selenium (Brazil nuts, seafood).
   - Limit processed foods, sugary snacks, and excessive intake of caffeine and alcohol, which can impair immune function.

2. **Hydration**:
   - Drink an adequate amount of water throughout the day to maintain hydration and support the body's natural detoxification processes.
   - Incorporate hydrating beverages such as herbal teas, coconut water, and homemade broths into daily routines.

3. **Regular Exercise**:
   - Engage in moderate-intensity exercise for at least 30 minutes most days of the week to promote circulation, reduce inflammation, and support immune function.
   - Choose activities that you enjoy, such as walking, jogging, cycling, yoga, or dancing, to make exercise a sustainable part of your lifestyle.

4. **Stress Management**:
   - Practice stress-reducing techniques such as deep breathing exercises, meditation, mindfulness, or progressive muscle relaxation to lower stress hormone levels and support immune function.
   - Incorporate stress-relieving activities into daily routines, such as spending time outdoors, listening to music, or engaging in creative hobbies.

5. **Adequate Sleep**:
   - Prioritize sleep hygiene practices, including establishing a consistent sleep schedule, creating a relaxing bedtime routine, and optimizing sleep environment conditions (e.g., comfortable bedding, dark room, moderate temperature).
   - Aim for 7-9 hours of quality sleep per night to support immune function, cognitive function, and overall well-being.

6. **Limit Exposure to Toxins**:
   - Minimize exposure to environmental toxins, such as air pollutants, household chemicals, and tobacco smoke, which can weaken the immune system and increase susceptibility to infections.
   - Use natural cleaning products, avoid smoking and secondhand smoke, and choose organic produce when possible to reduce toxin exposure.

By making these diet and lifestyle changes, individuals can strengthen their immune system, enhance overall health, and reduce the risk of contracting colds, flu, and other infections. Consistency and balance are key to maintaining long-term immune resilience and well-being.

Hygiene Practices to Prevent Cold and Flu

1. **Frequent Handwashing**:
   - Wash hands with soap and water for at least 20 seconds, especially after coughing, sneezing, using the restroom, or touching commonly-touched surfaces.
   - Use hand sanitizer containing at least 60% alcohol if soap and water are not available.

2. **Avoid Touching Face**:
   - Refrain from touching eyes, nose, and mouth with unwashed hands, as these are common entry points for viruses.
   - Use a tissue or elbow to cover the mouth and nose when coughing or sneezing to prevent the spread of respiratory droplets.

3. **Disinfect Frequently-Touched Surfaces**:
   - Regularly clean and disinfect high-touch surfaces such as doorknobs, light switches, countertops, and electronic devices using EPA-approved disinfectants.
   - Pay particular attention to shared surfaces in communal areas and workspaces.

4. **Practice Respiratory Etiquette**:
   - Cover mouth and nose with a tissue or elbow when coughing or sneezing to contain respiratory droplets and prevent the spread of viruses.
   - Dispose of used tissues immediately and wash hands thoroughly afterward.

5. **Maintain Distance**:
   - Practice social distancing by staying at least 6 feet away from individuals who are sick or showing symptoms of illness.
   - Avoid close contact, including handshakes and hugs, with individuals who may be contagious.

6. **Use Personal Protective Equipment (PPE)**:
   - Wear a mask or face covering in public settings, especially when social distancing is not possible, to reduce the transmission of respiratory droplets.
   - Replace masks regularly and wash reusable masks after each use.

7. **Promote Hygiene in Shared Spaces**:
   - Encourage cleanliness and hygiene practices in shared spaces such as schools, workplaces, and public transportation.
   - Provide hand sanitizer and tissues in accessible locations and encourage regular handwashing among individuals.

8. **Stay Home When Sick**:
   - If experiencing symptoms of cold or flu, stay home from work, school, and other public places to prevent the spread of illness to others.
   - Follow local health guidelines and recommendations for when it is safe to return to normal activities.

By incorporating these hygiene practices into daily routines, individuals can minimize the risk of contracting and spreading colds, flu, and other respiratory infections, creating a healthier environment for themselves and others.

Chapter 2

Herbal Remedies

1. **Echinacea (Echinacea purpurea):**
   - Known for its immune-boosting properties, echinacea is often used to reduce the severity and duration of cold symptoms.
   - Available in various forms, including capsules, tablets, tinctures, and teas.
   - Best taken at the onset of symptoms for maximum effectiveness.

2. **Elderberry (Sambucus nigra):**
   - Elderberry syrup is a popular remedy for colds and flu due to its antiviral and immune-stimulating effects.
   - Rich in antioxidants, elderberry can help reduce inflammation and promote respiratory health.
   - Available as syrup, capsules, and lozenges.

3. **Garlic (Allium sativum):**
   - Garlic has natural antimicrobial properties that can help fight off infections and boost immune function.
   - Consuming raw garlic or garlic supplements may help prevent and alleviate cold and flu symptoms.

- Incorporate garlic into meals or take garlic supplements for best results.

4. **Ginger (Zingiber officinale)**:
- Ginger has anti-inflammatory and antiviral properties that can help alleviate symptoms of colds and flu, including sore throat and congestion.
- Drink ginger tea, chew on raw ginger, or add ginger to soups, stir-fries, and smoothies for relief.
- Ginger supplements are also available for convenience.

5. **Peppermint (Mentha piperita)**:
- Peppermint contains menthol, which can help soothe sore throat, reduce coughing, and relieve congestion.
- Drink peppermint tea or inhale peppermint essential oil vapor for respiratory relief.
- Peppermint lozenges and syrups are also available for symptom relief.

6. **Licorice Root (Glycyrrhiza glabra)**:
- Licorice root has antiviral and expectorant properties that can help alleviate coughs, sore throat, and respiratory congestion.
- Drink licorice root tea or take licorice root supplements as directed for respiratory support.

- Avoid licorice root if you have high blood pressure or are pregnant.

7. **Oregano (Origanum vulgare)**:
   - Oregano contains compounds such as carvacrol and thymol, which have antimicrobial and immune-boosting effects.
   - Drink oregano tea, use oregano essential oil in steam inhalation, or add fresh or dried oregano to meals for respiratory support.

8. **Turmeric (Curcuma longa)**:
   - Turmeric contains curcumin, a compound with anti-inflammatory and antioxidant properties that can help alleviate symptoms of colds and flu.
   - Drink turmeric tea, add turmeric to curries and soups, or take turmeric supplements for immune support and symptom relief.

Before using herbal remedies, consult with a healthcare professional, especially if you have any underlying health conditions or are taking medications, to ensure safety and effectiveness.

Echinacea: Benefits and Usage

Echinacea, derived from the purple coneflower plant (Echinacea purpurea), is renowned for its immune-boosting properties and has been traditionally used to prevent and alleviate symptoms of colds, flu, and other respiratory infections. Here are its benefits and usage guidelines:

1. **Immune Support**:
   - Echinacea stimulates the immune system by increasing the production and activity of white blood cells, which play a crucial role in fighting off infections.
   - It contains compounds such as alkylamides, polysaccharides, and flavonoids that have immune-enhancing effects.

2. **Reduced Severity and Duration of Symptoms**:
   - Studies suggest that echinacea may help reduce the severity and duration of cold symptoms when taken at the onset of illness.
   - It can alleviate symptoms such as sore throat, congestion, coughing, and fatigue, helping individuals recover more quickly.

3. **Antiviral and Antioxidant Properties**:
   - Echinacea exhibits antiviral properties that can inhibit the replication of cold and flu viruses, helping to prevent the spread of infection.
   - It also has antioxidant properties that protect cells from damage caused by free radicals, promoting overall health and well-being.

4. **Anti-inflammatory Effects**:
   - Echinacea has anti-inflammatory effects that can help reduce inflammation in the respiratory tract, easing symptoms such as nasal congestion and throat irritation.

5. **Usage Guidelines**:
   - Echinacea is available in various forms, including capsules, tablets, tinctures, and teas.
   - It is best taken at the onset of cold symptoms for maximum effectiveness.
   - Follow the dosage instructions provided on the product label or consult with a healthcare professional for personalized recommendations.
   - Avoid prolonged use of echinacea, as it may decrease its effectiveness over time.
   - Individuals with autoimmune disorders, allergies to plants in the Asteraceae family (such as ragweed), or certain medical conditions should

consult with a healthcare professional before using echinacea.

Overall, echinacea can be a valuable natural remedy for supporting immune function and alleviating symptoms of colds and flu. When used appropriately, it can help individuals boost their defenses against respiratory infections and promote faster recovery.

Elderberry Syrup: An Immune-Boosting Elixir

Elderberry syrup, derived from the berries of the elder tree (Sambucus nigra), is renowned for its immune-boosting properties and has been used for centuries to prevent and alleviate symptoms of colds, flu, and other respiratory infections. Here's an overview of its benefits and usage:

1. **Immune Support**:
   - Elderberries are rich in vitamins A, B, and C, as well as flavonoids and antioxidants, which help strengthen the immune system and enhance its ability to fight off infections.

- The anthocyanins found in elderberries have been shown to stimulate the production of cytokines, proteins that regulate immune response.

2. **Antiviral Properties**:
   - Elderberry syrup contains compounds that have been found to inhibit the replication of cold and flu viruses, preventing them from spreading and causing illness.
   - Studies have shown that elderberry syrup can help reduce the duration and severity of cold and flu symptoms when taken at the onset of illness.

3. **Anti-inflammatory Effects**:
   - Elderberries have anti-inflammatory properties that can help reduce inflammation in the respiratory tract, alleviating symptoms such as nasal congestion, sore throat, and coughing.

4. **Rich in Antioxidants**:
   - Elderberries are packed with antioxidants, such as quercetin and rutin, which help protect cells from damage caused by free radicals and support overall health and well-being.

5. **Usage Guidelines**:
   - Elderberry syrup is available commercially or can be made at home using dried elderberries, water, and honey or other sweeteners.
   - It is typically recommended to take elderberry syrup at the onset of cold or flu symptoms for maximum effectiveness.
   - Follow the dosage instructions provided on the product label or consult with a healthcare professional for personalized recommendations.
   - Elderberry syrup can be taken alone or mixed with water, juice, or tea for a pleasant and soothing beverage.
   - Individuals with certain medical conditions or allergies should consult with a healthcare professional before using elderberry syrup.

Overall, elderberry syrup is a delicious and effective immune-boosting elixir that can help individuals prevent and alleviate symptoms of colds, flu, and other respiratory infections. When used as part of a healthy lifestyle, it can support immune function and promote overall well-being.

Garlic: Nature's Antibiotic

Garlic (Allium sativum) has been revered for centuries for its potent medicinal properties, earning it the nickname "nature's antibiotic." Here's an overview of its benefits and usage:

1. **Antimicrobial Properties**:
   - Garlic contains allicin, a sulfur compound with powerful antimicrobial properties that can help fight off bacteria, viruses, fungi, and parasites.
   - Allicin is formed when garlic is crushed, chopped, or chewed, releasing its therapeutic benefits.

2. **Immune Support**:
   - Garlic stimulates the immune system by increasing the production and activity of white blood cells, which play a crucial role in defending the body against infections.
   - Regular consumption of garlic may help prevent common colds, flu, and other respiratory infections.

3. **Cardiovascular Health**:
   - Garlic has been shown to lower blood pressure, reduce cholesterol levels, and improve blood circulation, thereby reducing the risk of heart disease and stroke.

- Its anti-inflammatory properties may also help prevent the development of atherosclerosis and improve overall cardiovascular function.

4. **Antioxidant Effects**:
   - Garlic is rich in antioxidants, such as selenium and vitamin C, which help protect cells from oxidative damage caused by free radicals.
   - Antioxidants play a key role in reducing inflammation, boosting immunity, and promoting overall health and longevity.

5. **Usage Guidelines**:
   - Incorporate fresh garlic into meals regularly to reap its health benefits. Raw garlic is the most potent, but cooked garlic still retains many of its medicinal properties.
   - Garlic supplements, including garlic capsules, tablets, and extracts, are also available for those who prefer a more convenient option.
   - Crush or chop garlic and let it sit for a few minutes before consuming to maximize the formation of allicin.
   - Start with small amounts of garlic and gradually increase intake to avoid digestive discomfort or strong odor.

6. **Precautions**:
   - Some individuals may be allergic to garlic or experience gastrointestinal upset, heartburn, or bad breath with excessive consumption.
   - Garlic may interact with certain medications, including blood thinners and HIV/AIDS medications, so consult with a healthcare professional before using garlic supplements.

Overall, garlic is a versatile and potent natural remedy that can help support immune function, promote cardiovascular health, and ward off infections. Incorporating garlic into your diet regularly can contribute to a healthier and more resilient body.

Ginger: Soothing and Anti-inflammatory Properties

Ginger (Zingiber officinale) is renowned for its soothing and anti-inflammatory properties, making it a popular natural remedy for various ailments. Here's an overview of its benefits and usage:

1. **Anti-inflammatory Effects**:
   - Ginger contains bioactive compounds such as gingerol, shogaol, and paradol, which have potent anti-inflammatory properties.
   - These compounds help reduce inflammation in the body, alleviating symptoms of conditions such as arthritis, muscle soreness, and inflammatory bowel disease.

2. **Digestive Support**:
   - Ginger has been used for centuries to aid digestion and relieve gastrointestinal discomfort.
   - It helps stimulate saliva production, promote gastric motility, and reduce nausea and vomiting, making it particularly effective for motion sickness, morning sickness, and chemotherapy-induced nausea.

3. **Immune Boosting**:
   - Ginger contains antioxidants that help strengthen the immune system and protect against oxidative stress.
   - Regular consumption of ginger may help reduce the risk of infections, including colds, flu, and respiratory illnesses.

4. **Soothing Properties**:
   - Ginger has a warming and soothing effect on the body, making it beneficial for alleviating symptoms of colds, flu, and respiratory congestion.
   - It can help relieve sore throat, coughing, and nasal congestion by promoting circulation and loosening mucus.

5. **Pain Relief**:
   - Ginger has analgesic properties that can help reduce pain and discomfort associated with headaches, menstrual cramps, and muscle tension.
   - It may be as effective as conventional pain relievers in some cases, with fewer side effects.

6. **Usage Guidelines**:
   - Incorporate fresh ginger into meals by grating or slicing it and adding it to stir-fries, soups, teas, and smoothies.
   - Drink ginger tea by steeping fresh ginger slices or ginger tea bags in hot water for a soothing beverage.
   - Chew on a small piece of fresh ginger or suck on ginger candies to alleviate nausea and indigestion.
   - Ginger supplements, including capsules, tablets, and extracts, are also available for those who prefer a more concentrated dose.

7. **Precautions**:
   - While ginger is generally safe for most people, excessive consumption may cause digestive upset or interact with certain medications, including blood thinners and diabetes medications.
   - Pregnant women should consult with a healthcare professional before using ginger supplements, especially in large amounts.

Overall, ginger is a versatile and effective natural remedy that can help soothe inflammation, aid digestion, boost immunity, and alleviate symptoms of various health conditions. Incorporating ginger into your daily routine can promote overall health and well-being.

Chapter 3

Vitamins and Supplements

1. **Vitamin C**:
   - Supports immune function and helps reduce the duration and severity of cold symptoms.
   - Found in citrus fruits, strawberries, kiwi, bell peppers, and supplements.

2. **Zinc**:
   - Plays a role in immune function and may help shorten the duration of colds when taken at the onset of symptoms.
   - Found in shellfish, meat, nuts, seeds, and supplements.

3. **Vitamin D**:
   - Supports immune function and may reduce the risk of respiratory infections.
   - Obtained from sunlight exposure, fatty fish, fortified dairy products, and supplements.

4. **Echinacea**:
   - Herbal remedy known for its immune-boosting properties and ability to reduce cold symptoms.
   - Available in various forms, including capsules, tablets, tinctures, and teas.

5. **Elderberry**:
   - Rich in antioxidants and flavonoids, elderberry may help boost immunity and reduce the severity and duration of cold and flu symptoms.
   - Available as syrup, capsules, and lozenges.

6. **Garlic**:
   - Contains compounds with antimicrobial and immune-boosting properties that may help prevent and alleviate cold and flu symptoms.
   - Consumed raw, cooked, or in supplement form.

7. **Probiotics**:
   - Beneficial bacteria that support gut health and may help strengthen the immune system.
   - Found in yogurt, kefir, sauerkraut, and supplements.

8. **Echinacea**:
   - Herbal remedy known for its immune-boosting properties and ability to reduce cold symptoms.
   - Available in various forms, including capsules, tablets, tinctures, and teas.

9. **Elderberry**:
   - Rich in antioxidants and flavonoids, elderberry may help boost immunity and reduce the severity and duration of cold and flu symptoms.

- Available as syrup, capsules, and lozenges.

10. **Garlic**:
   - Contains compounds with antimicrobial and immune-boosting properties that may help prevent and alleviate cold and flu symptoms.
   - Consumed raw, cooked, or in supplement form.

11. **Probiotics**:
   - Beneficial bacteria that support gut health and may help strengthen the immune system.
   - Found in yogurt, kefir, sauerkraut, and supplements.

12. **Omega-3 Fatty Acids**:
   - Have anti-inflammatory properties that may help reduce inflammation and support immune function.
   - Found in fatty fish, flaxseeds, chia seeds, and supplements.

13. **Vitamin E**:
   - An antioxidant that helps protect cells from damage and supports immune function.
   - Found in nuts, seeds, vegetable oils, and supplements.

14. **Vitamin A**:
   - Essential for immune function and maintaining healthy mucous membranes.
   - Found in liver, eggs, dairy products, and supplements.

When considering supplements, it's important to consult with a healthcare professional to determine the appropriate dosage and ensure compatibility with other medications or medical conditions. Additionally, obtaining nutrients from a balanced diet is ideal whenever possible.

Vitamin C: Immune Support and Symptom Relief

Vitamin C, also known as ascorbic acid, is a powerful antioxidant that plays a crucial role in supporting immune function and alleviating symptoms of respiratory infections like colds and flu. Here's an overview of its benefits and usage:

1. **Immune Support**:
   - Vitamin C enhances the function of various immune cells, including neutrophils, lymphocytes, and phagocytes, which help defend the body against infections.

- It stimulates the production of white blood cells and antibodies, essential components of the immune system's response to pathogens.

2. **Antioxidant Properties**:
   - Vitamin C is a potent antioxidant that helps protect cells from oxidative stress caused by free radicals.
   - By neutralizing free radicals, vitamin C helps reduce inflammation and supports overall immune function.

3. **Reduced Duration and Severity of Symptoms**:
   - Studies have shown that vitamin C supplementation can help reduce the duration and severity of cold symptoms.
   - It may help alleviate symptoms such as nasal congestion, sore throat, coughing, and fatigue, allowing individuals to recover more quickly.

4. **Enhanced Collagen Production**:
   - Vitamin C is essential for the synthesis of collagen, a structural protein that supports the skin, mucous membranes, and connective tissues.
   - Adequate intake of vitamin C promotes wound healing and strengthens the body's natural barriers against pathogens.

5. **Usage Guidelines**:
   - Vitamin C is found naturally in fruits and vegetables, including citrus fruits, strawberries, kiwi, bell peppers, and leafy greens.
   - It is also available in supplemental form, including capsules, tablets, powders, and chewable tablets.
   - During cold and flu season or when experiencing symptoms of respiratory infections, consider increasing vitamin C intake through diet and supplements.
   - Follow the dosage instructions provided on the product label or consult with a healthcare professional for personalized recommendations.
   - Vitamin C supplements are generally safe for most people when taken within recommended doses, but excessive intake may cause digestive upset in some individuals.

6. **Precautions**:
   - Individuals with certain medical conditions, such as kidney stones or iron overload disorders, should consult with a healthcare professional before taking high-dose vitamin C supplements.
   - Pregnant and breastfeeding women should also seek medical advice before supplementing with vitamin C to ensure safety for themselves and their baby.

Overall, vitamin C is a valuable nutrient for supporting immune function, reducing the severity and duration of cold symptoms, and promoting overall health and well-being. Incorporating vitamin C-rich foods into your diet and considering supplementation when needed can help optimize immune health and resilience against respiratory infections.

Zinc: Shortening Cold Duration and Reducing Severity

Zinc is a mineral that plays a crucial role in various physiological processes, including immune function. Here's an overview of how zinc can help shorten the duration and reduce the severity of colds:

1. **Immune Support**:
   - Zinc is essential for the proper functioning of immune cells, including T cells, B cells, and natural killer cells, which help fight off infections.
   - Adequate zinc levels are necessary for maintaining a robust immune response and reducing susceptibility to respiratory infections like colds.

2. **Antiviral Properties**:
   - Zinc has been shown to have direct antiviral effects against cold-causing viruses, such as rhinoviruses and coronaviruses.
   - It inhibits viral replication and may help prevent the spread of viruses within the body, reducing the severity and duration of cold symptoms.

3. **Reduced Cold Duration**:
   - Studies have found that zinc supplementation can help shorten the duration of colds when taken within 24 hours of symptom onset.
   - Zinc lozenges or syrup formulations containing zinc acetate or zinc gluconate are commonly used for this purpose.

4. **Symptom Relief**:
   - Zinc may also help alleviate symptoms of colds, such as nasal congestion, sore throat, coughing, and sneezing.
   - It has mucolytic properties that can help loosen mucus and improve respiratory function, making breathing easier.

5. **Usage Guidelines**:
   - Zinc is found naturally in various foods, including meat, shellfish, nuts, seeds, dairy products, and whole grains.

- Zinc supplements are available in different forms, including tablets, capsules, lozenges, and syrups.
- When using zinc lozenges or syrup for cold relief, it's important to start taking them at the first sign of symptoms and continue for the duration recommended on the product label.
- Follow the dosage instructions provided on the product label or consult with a healthcare professional for personalized recommendations.
- Excessive intake of zinc supplements can lead to adverse effects, such as nausea, vomiting, and diarrhea, so it's essential to stick to recommended doses.

6. **Precautions**:
   - Individuals with certain medical conditions, such as Wilson's disease or hemochromatosis, should consult with a healthcare professional before supplementing with zinc.
   - Pregnant and breastfeeding women should also seek medical advice before using zinc supplements to ensure safety for themselves and their baby.

Overall, zinc is a valuable nutrient for supporting immune function and reducing the severity and duration of cold symptoms. Incorporating zinc-rich foods into your diet and considering supplementation when needed can help enhance immune health and resilience against respiratory infections.

Vitamin D: Enhancing Immune Function

Vitamin D is a fat-soluble vitamin that plays a crucial role in supporting immune function and overall health. Here's an overview of how vitamin D can enhance immune function:

1. **Regulating Immune Response**:
   - Vitamin D plays a role in modulating the innate and adaptive immune responses, helping to maintain immune homeostasis and prevent excessive inflammation.
   - It enhances the function of various immune cells, including macrophages, T cells, and B cells, which play key roles in recognizing and eliminating pathogens.

2. **Antimicrobial Properties**:
   - Vitamin D has been shown to have direct antimicrobial effects against a wide range of pathogens, including bacteria, viruses, and fungi.
   - It helps stimulate the production of antimicrobial peptides, such as cathelicidin and

defensins, which can destroy invading microorganisms and protect against infections.

3. **Reducing Risk of Respiratory Infections**:
   - Adequate vitamin D levels have been associated with a reduced risk of respiratory infections, including colds, flu, and pneumonia.
   - Vitamin D deficiency has been linked to an increased susceptibility to respiratory illnesses, especially during the winter months when sunlight exposure is limited.

4. **Anti-inflammatory Effects**:
   - Vitamin D helps regulate the production of pro-inflammatory cytokines, reducing inflammation and promoting immune tolerance.
   - By modulating immune responses, vitamin D may help prevent chronic inflammatory conditions and autoimmune diseases.

5. **Usage Guidelines**:
   - Vitamin D is synthesized by the skin upon exposure to sunlight, but it can also be obtained from dietary sources and supplements.
   - Foods rich in vitamin D include fatty fish (e.g., salmon, mackerel, tuna), egg yolks, fortified dairy products, and fortified cereals.

- Vitamin D supplements are available in various forms, including capsules, tablets, and liquid drops.
- The recommended daily allowance (RDA) for vitamin D varies depending on age, sex, and other factors. It's generally recommended to aim for blood levels of 25-hydroxyvitamin D (the circulating form of vitamin D) between 30-50 ng/mL for optimal health.
- Individuals with limited sun exposure, darker skin tones, older adults, and those with certain medical conditions may benefit from vitamin D supplementation.

6. **Precautions**:
- While vitamin D toxicity is rare, excessive intake of vitamin D supplements can lead to hypercalcemia (elevated blood calcium levels) and other adverse effects.
- It's important to monitor vitamin D levels regularly and consult with a healthcare professional for personalized supplementation recommendations.

Overall, vitamin D plays a critical role in enhancing immune function and protecting against respiratory infections. Ensuring adequate vitamin D intake through sunlight exposure, dietary sources, and supplements can help support immune health and overall well-being.

Chapter 4

Hydration and Warmth

1. **Hydration**:
   - Drinking an adequate amount of water is essential for maintaining hydration levels, supporting overall health, and facilitating the body's natural detoxification processes.
   - Proper hydration helps keep mucous membranes in the respiratory tract moist, which can help prevent irritation and discomfort associated with colds and flu.
   - Aim to drink at least 8-10 glasses of water per day, and increase fluid intake when experiencing symptoms of respiratory infections to prevent dehydration.

2. **Warm Liquids**:
   - Consuming warm liquids such as herbal teas, broths, soups, and warm water with lemon can provide soothing relief for sore throat, nasal congestion, and coughing.
   - Warm liquids help hydrate the body, loosen mucus, and alleviate respiratory symptoms by promoting relaxation and improving circulation.
   - Adding ingredients like ginger, honey, lemon, and cinnamon to warm beverages can enhance their

therapeutic properties and provide additional immune support.

3. **Moisture**:
   - Using a humidifier in the home, especially during the winter months when indoor air tends to be dry, can help maintain optimal humidity levels and prevent dryness in the respiratory tract.
   - Moist air can soothe irritated nasal passages, reduce congestion, and promote more comfortable breathing, particularly for individuals with colds or flu.

4. **Warmth**:
   - Keeping the body warm and maintaining a comfortable ambient temperature is important for supporting immune function and preventing heat loss during periods of illness.
   - Dressing in layers, using blankets, and staying indoors in a heated environment can help maintain body temperature and promote comfort and relaxation.
   - Avoiding exposure to cold temperatures and drafts can help prevent further stress on the immune system and exacerbation of symptoms.

5. **Steam Inhalation**:
   - Inhaling steam from a bowl of hot water or a steam inhaler can help moisturize nasal passages, clear congestion, and provide relief from sinus pressure and headache.
   - Adding essential oils such as eucalyptus, peppermint, or tea tree oil to the steam can enhance its therapeutic effects and promote respiratory comfort.

6. **Warm Baths**:
   - Taking a warm bath with Epsom salts, essential oils, or bath bombs can help relax muscles, reduce stress, and promote overall well-being during times of illness.
   - Adding soothing ingredients like oatmeal or baking soda to the bathwater can help alleviate skin irritation and promote hydration.

By prioritizing hydration and warmth, individuals can support their immune system, alleviate symptoms of respiratory infections, and promote overall comfort and well-being during cold and flu season. Incorporating warm liquids, moisture, and relaxation techniques into daily routines can help enhance immune resilience and facilitate recovery from illness.

Importance of Adequate Hydration

1. **Optimal Body Functioning**:
   - Adequate hydration is essential for maintaining optimal body functioning. Water plays a critical role in nearly every bodily process, including digestion, circulation, temperature regulation, and waste elimination.

2. **Cellular Health**:
   - Water is the primary component of cells and tissues in the body. Proper hydration ensures that cells receive essential nutrients and oxygen while removing waste products and toxins, promoting cellular health and function.

3. **Hydration of Mucous Membranes**:
   - Adequate hydration helps keep mucous membranes in the respiratory tract, digestive system, and urinary tract moist and lubricated. Moist mucous membranes are better able to trap pathogens and prevent infections.

4. **Supports Immune Function**:
   - Staying hydrated is crucial for supporting immune function. Water helps transport immune cells throughout the body and facilitates the

elimination of pathogens and toxins, reducing the risk of illness and infection.

5. **Detoxification**:
   - Hydration is essential for proper detoxification processes in the body. Water helps flush out toxins, metabolic waste products, and other harmful substances through urine, sweat, and bowel movements, promoting overall health and well-being.

6. **Cognitive Function**:
   - Dehydration can impair cognitive function, leading to decreased concentration, fatigue, and mood disturbances. Staying hydrated helps maintain mental clarity, alertness, and cognitive performance.

7. **Physical Performance**:
   - Proper hydration is crucial for athletic performance and physical endurance. Dehydration can lead to muscle cramps, fatigue, and decreased exercise performance. Drinking water before, during, and after physical activity helps maintain hydration levels and optimize performance.

8. **Regulation of Body Temperature**:
   - Water helps regulate body temperature by facilitating sweat production and evaporation, which helps cool the body during periods of heat stress or physical exertion.

9. **Prevention of Dehydration**:
   - Dehydration occurs when the body loses more water than it takes in, leading to symptoms such as thirst, dry mouth, headache, dizziness, and dark urine. Chronic dehydration can have serious health consequences and should be avoided by maintaining adequate fluid intake.

10. **Overall Health and Well-being**:
    - Adequate hydration is essential for overall health and well-being. It supports proper organ function, maintains electrolyte balance, and promotes vitality and longevity.

In conclusion, staying adequately hydrated is crucial for maintaining optimal health, supporting immune function, promoting detoxification, and enhancing physical and cognitive performance. It's essential to drink water regularly throughout the day and pay attention to thirst cues to ensure proper hydration and well-being.

Hot Liquids: Herbal Teas, Broths, and Soups

1. **Herbal Teas**:
   - Herbal teas, such as chamomile, ginger, peppermint, and echinacea, offer soothing relief for cold and flu symptoms.
   - Chamomile tea calms nerves and aids sleep.
   - Ginger tea reduces inflammation and relieves nausea.
   - Peppermint tea eases congestion and aids digestion.
   - Echinacea tea boosts immunity and reduces cold severity.

2. **Broths**:
   - Chicken or vegetable broths are hydrating and nutrient-rich, providing electrolytes, vitamins, and minerals.
   - Broths soothe sore throats, replenish nutrients, and support immune function.
   - Warm broth comforts and nourishes during illness.

3. **Soups**:
   - Warm soups with vegetables, protein, and herbs are comforting and healing meals.
   - Chicken noodle soup hydrates, delivers nutrients, and reduces inflammation.

- Adding garlic, onions, and turmeric enhances immune support and respiratory health.

4. **Warm Water with Lemon and Honey**:
   - Warm water with lemon and honey soothes sore throats and coughs.
   - Lemon provides vitamin C and antioxidants, while honey offers antimicrobial properties.
   - Adding ginger or cinnamon enhances flavor and immune benefits.

5. **Usage Tips**:
   - Drink hot liquids regularly throughout the day for hydration and nourishment.
   - Opt for low-sodium or homemade broths and soups for optimal nutrition.
   - Experiment with herbs, spices, and ingredients to tailor hot liquids to personal preferences and health needs.

Incorporating herbal teas, broths, and soups into your diet provides hydration, comfort, and nutritional support during colds, flu, and respiratory infections. These beverages alleviate symptoms and promote immune function, aiding in faster recovery.

Chapter 5

Steam Therapy and Inhalation

1. **Steam Inhalation**:
   - Steam inhalation involves inhaling warm, moist air to help relieve congestion and respiratory symptoms.
   - Boil water in a pot and remove from heat. Lean over the pot with a towel draped over your head to trap the steam, then inhale deeply through your nose for several minutes.
   - Alternatively, use a steam inhaler or facial steamer for convenience and targeted delivery of steam to the nasal passages and throat.

2. **Benefits**:
   - Moisture from steam helps hydrate and soothe irritated nasal passages, throat, and bronchial tubes, providing relief from congestion, sinus pressure, and coughing.
   - Steam helps loosen mucus and phlegm, making it easier to expel from the respiratory tract and improving breathing.
   - Inhaling steam can also help reduce inflammation and irritation in the airways, providing comfort and promoting relaxation.

3. **Additives**:
   - Adding essential oils such as eucalyptus, peppermint, or tea tree oil to the steam can enhance its therapeutic effects.
   - These oils have antimicrobial, decongestant, and anti-inflammatory properties that can further alleviate respiratory symptoms and promote healing.

4. **Usage Tips**:
   - Perform steam inhalation sessions 2-3 times per day or as needed to relieve symptoms.
   - Be cautious to avoid burns from hot steam, especially with young children or individuals with sensitive skin.
   - Keep a safe distance from the source of steam to prevent accidental burns or scalding.
   - If using essential oils, start with a small amount and dilute properly to avoid irritation or allergic reactions.
   - Steam therapy can be combined with other home remedies such as herbal teas, hydration, and rest for enhanced symptom relief and faster recovery from respiratory infections.

Incorporating steam therapy and inhalation into your self-care routine can provide effective relief from congestion, sinus pressure, and respiratory discomfort associated with colds, flu, and other respiratory infections. This natural remedy is easy to use and can be customized with essential oils for added therapeutic benefits.

Steam Inhalation with Essential Oils

1. **Preparation**:
   - Boil water in a pot or use a facial steamer to produce steam. Remove from heat and transfer the hot water to a heat-resistant bowl.
   - Add 2-3 drops of essential oil to the hot water. Popular choices include eucalyptus, peppermint, tea tree, lavender, and rosemary.

2. **Inhalation Technique**:
   - Position yourself comfortably over the bowl of hot water, ensuring a safe distance to avoid burns.
   - Close your eyes and drape a towel over your head to create a tent, trapping the steam inside.
   - Inhale deeply and slowly through your nose, allowing the aromatic steam to penetrate your nasal passages and respiratory tract.

3. **Benefits of Essential Oils**:
   - Eucalyptus oil: Acts as a decongestant, relieving nasal congestion and sinus pressure. It also has

antimicrobial properties that can help fight off respiratory infections.

- Peppermint oil: Provides a cooling sensation and helps clear nasal passages. It has antiviral and anti-inflammatory properties that can alleviate respiratory symptoms.
- Tea tree oil: Known for its antimicrobial and immune-boosting properties, tea tree oil can help combat respiratory infections and soothe inflamed airways.
- Lavender oil: Calming and relaxing, lavender oil can help reduce stress and promote restful sleep, which is beneficial during illness.
- Rosemary oil: Contains compounds that support respiratory health and may help relieve coughing and congestion.

4. **Safety Considerations**:
   - Use caution when handling essential oils, as they are potent and can cause skin irritation or allergic reactions in some individuals. Always dilute them properly before use.
   - Start with a low concentration of essential oil and adjust based on personal preference and tolerance.
   - Keep essential oils out of reach of children and pets, and avoid contact with eyes and mucous membranes.

- If you experience any adverse reactions or discomfort, discontinue use immediately and seek medical advice if necessary.

5. **Frequency and Duration**:
   - Perform steam inhalation with essential oils 1-2 times per day or as needed to relieve respiratory symptoms.
   - Each session can last for 5-10 minutes, but avoid prolonged exposure to steam to prevent dehydration or skin irritation.

Using steam inhalation with essential oils is a natural and effective way to relieve congestion, sinus pressure, and respiratory discomfort during colds, flu, and other respiratory infections. It harnesses the therapeutic benefits of both steam and essential oils to promote respiratory health and well-being.

Nasal Irrigation with Saline Solution

1. **Preparation**:
   - Prepare a saline solution by mixing 1 teaspoon of non-iodized salt (such as sea salt or kosher salt) with 2 cups of lukewarm distilled or sterile water.

Ensure that the water is properly sterilized to prevent infection.

- Optionally, add a pinch of baking soda to the saline solution to help soothe the nasal passages and reduce irritation.

2. **Nasal Irrigation Technique**:
   - Stand over a sink or basin and tilt your head slightly forward.
   - Gently insert the tip of a neti pot, squeeze bottle, or nasal irrigation device into one nostril.
   - Tilt the device so that the saline solution flows into your nostril and out through the opposite nostril. Breathe through your mouth during the process.
   - Allow the saline solution to flow freely through your nasal passages, flushing out mucus, allergens, and irritants. Avoid swallowing the saline solution.
   - Repeat the process with the other nostril.

3. **Benefits of Nasal Irrigation**:
   - Clears nasal passages: Nasal irrigation helps remove excess mucus, allergens, and irritants from the nasal passages, providing relief from congestion and sinus pressure.
   - Reduces inflammation: Saline solution helps soothe inflamed nasal tissues and reduce swelling, promoting easier breathing.

- Moisturizes nasal passages: Nasal irrigation moisturizes dry nasal passages, relieving discomfort and preventing further irritation.
- Promotes sinus health: Regular nasal irrigation can help prevent sinus infections and promote overall sinus health by keeping the nasal passages clean and clear.

4. **Safety Considerations**:
   - Use only sterile or distilled water for nasal irrigation to avoid introducing harmful bacteria or organisms into the nasal passages.
   - Ensure that the saline solution is properly mixed to the correct concentration to prevent irritation.
   - Avoid nasal irrigation if you have a severe nasal obstruction, a deviated septum, or a recent nosebleed, as it may worsen these conditions.
   - Clean and disinfect the neti pot or nasal irrigation device after each use to prevent bacterial growth and contamination.

5. **Frequency and Duration**:
   - Nasal irrigation can be performed 1-2 times per day or as needed to relieve nasal congestion and sinus symptoms.
   - It is safe for regular use and can be incorporated into your daily nasal hygiene routine, especially during colds, allergies, or sinusitis.

Nasal irrigation with saline solution is a safe and effective method for relieving nasal congestion, sinus pressure, and other nasal symptoms associated with colds, allergies, and sinus infections. It helps clear the nasal passages, reduce inflammation, and promote sinus health, providing natural relief from nasal discomfort.

Chapter 6

Rest and Sleep

1. **Importance of Rest**:
   - Rest is essential for allowing the body to recover and heal during times of illness, including colds and flu.
   - Taking time to rest helps conserve energy and resources that can be redirected towards fighting off infections and supporting immune function.

2. **Promotes Healing**:
   - Adequate rest allows the body to focus its resources on combating pathogens and repairing damaged tissues, accelerating the healing process.
   - Restorative sleep is particularly important for immune function, as it enhances the production of immune cells and promotes immune surveillance against pathogens.

3. **Reduces Symptoms**:
   - Rest can help alleviate symptoms associated with colds and flu, such as fatigue, body aches, and fever.
   - Taking time to rest allows the body to recuperate and recover from the physical stress of illness, resulting in improved comfort and well-being.

4. **Supports Immune Function**:
   - Chronic sleep deprivation can weaken the immune system and increase susceptibility to infections.
   - Prioritizing adequate sleep during illness helps support immune function and optimize the body's ability to fight off pathogens.

5. **Tips for Rest and Sleep**:
   - Listen to your body's signals and prioritize rest when feeling fatigued or unwell.
   - Create a comfortable and conducive sleep environment by ensuring a cool, dark, and quiet room.
   - Establish a regular sleep schedule and aim for 7-9 hours of quality sleep per night.
   - Practice relaxation techniques such as deep breathing, meditation, or gentle stretching before bedtime to promote restful sleep.
   - Avoid caffeine, alcohol, and electronic devices close to bedtime, as they can interfere with sleep quality and duration.

6. **Napping**:
   - Short naps during the day can provide additional rest and rejuvenation, especially when feeling tired or run down.

- Aim for brief naps of 20-30 minutes to avoid disrupting nighttime sleep patterns.

7. **Seek Medical Attention**:
   - If symptoms persist or worsen despite adequate rest and self-care measures, consult a healthcare professional for further evaluation and treatment.

Incorporating rest and prioritizing sleep during illness is crucial for supporting the body's natural healing processes, reducing symptoms, and promoting overall recovery. By allowing the body to rest and recharge, individuals can enhance their resilience and shorten the duration of colds and flu.

The Healing Power of Rest

Rest is not merely a luxury but a vital component of the body's healing process, particularly during times of illness such as colds and flu. Here's how rest contributes to healing:

1. **Conservation of Energy**: When the body is fighting off an infection, it requires a significant amount of energy to mount an immune response. Resting allows the body to conserve energy that can

be redirected towards combating pathogens and supporting immune function.

2. **Cellular Repair and Regeneration**: During restful periods, the body prioritizes cellular repair and regeneration. This includes repairing damaged tissues, replenishing depleted energy stores, and removing waste products accumulated during the illness.

3. **Immune System Support**: Adequate rest plays a crucial role in supporting immune function. Sleep, in particular, is essential for the production of immune cells and the regulation of immune responses. By getting enough rest, the body can strengthen its defenses and more effectively fend off invading pathogens.

4. **Reduction of Inflammation**: Rest has been shown to reduce inflammation in the body, which is a common response to infection. By minimizing inflammation, rest can help alleviate symptoms such as sore throat, congestion, and body aches associated with colds and flu.

5. **Enhanced Recovery**: Restorative sleep, in particular, promotes enhanced recovery from illness. Quality sleep allows the body to enter

deeper stages of sleep where tissue repair, hormone regulation, and immune function optimization occur. This leads to faster recovery and improved overall well-being.

6. **Stress Reduction**: Resting also helps reduce stress levels, which can have a significant impact on immune function. High levels of stress hormones like cortisol can suppress immune activity, making it harder for the body to fight off infections. Taking time to rest and relax can counteract these effects and support immune health.

7. **Prevention of Complications**: By allowing the body to fully rest and recover from illness, individuals can reduce the risk of developing complications associated with colds and flu, such as secondary infections or prolonged illness.

In summary, rest is a fundamental aspect of the body's healing process. By prioritizing rest during illness, individuals can support their immune system, accelerate recovery, and reduce the severity of symptoms associated with colds and flu. Whether through adequate sleep, relaxation, or simply taking it easy, embracing the healing power of rest is essential for overall health and well-being.

Creating a comfortable sleeping environment is essential for promoting restful sleep, especially during times of illness such as colds and flu. Here are some tips to create an optimal sleeping environment:

1. **Temperature Control**:
   - Keep the bedroom temperature comfortably cool, between 60-67 degrees Fahrenheit (15-19 degrees Celsius), to promote restful sleep.
   - Use breathable bedding materials such as cotton sheets and blankets to help regulate body temperature and prevent overheating.

2. **Light Management**:
   - Keep the bedroom dark and conducive to sleep by using blackout curtains or blinds to block out unwanted light.
   - Minimize exposure to electronic devices with bright screens before bedtime, as the blue light emitted can disrupt the body's natural sleep-wake cycle.

3. **Noise Reduction**:
   - Minimize noise disruptions by using earplugs or white noise machines to block out unwanted sounds such as traffic, neighbors, or household noises.

- If noise is unavoidable, consider using a fan or soothing soundscape to mask disruptive noises and promote relaxation.

4. **Comfortable Bedding**:
- Invest in a comfortable mattress and pillows that provide adequate support and alignment for your body.
- Choose bedding with soft, breathable fabrics that feel comfortable against the skin and promote relaxation.

5. **Aromatherapy**:
- Use calming essential oils such as lavender, chamomile, or cedarwood to create a relaxing atmosphere in the bedroom.
- Diffuse essential oils or use a pillow spray to infuse the air with soothing scents that promote relaxation and sleep.

6. **Declutter and Organize**:
- Keep the bedroom clean, clutter-free, and organized to create a serene and calming environment conducive to sleep.
- Remove distractions such as work-related materials, electronic devices, and clutter from the bedroom to promote relaxation and reduce stress.

7. **Comforting Rituals**:
   - Establish a relaxing bedtime routine to signal to your body that it's time to wind down and prepare for sleep.
   - Engage in calming activities such as reading, gentle stretching, or taking a warm bath to promote relaxation and ease into sleep.

8. **Optimal Humidity**:
   - Maintain optimal humidity levels in the bedroom to prevent dry air that can lead to discomfort and disrupted sleep.
   - Use a humidifier or dehumidifier as needed to adjust humidity levels and create a comfortable sleeping environment.

By implementing these strategies, you can create a comfortable and soothing sleeping environment that promotes restful sleep and enhances your body's ability to recover from illness. Prioritizing sleep hygiene and creating a conducive sleep environment can help support overall health and well-being, especially during times of illness.

Chapter 7

Humidification

Humidification plays a crucial role in creating a comfortable and healthy sleeping environment, especially during times of illness like colds and flu. Here's how humidification can benefit sleep and overall well-being:

1. **Moisturizes Respiratory Tract**: Humidifiers add moisture to the air, helping to prevent dryness in the nasal passages, throat, and lungs. This can alleviate symptoms such as sore throat, nasal congestion, and coughing, making it easier to breathe and sleep comfortably.

2. **Relieves Congestion**: Increased humidity can help loosen mucus and congestion in the respiratory tract, facilitating easier breathing and reducing discomfort associated with nasal congestion and sinus pressure.

3. **Promotes Comfortable Sleep**: Optimal humidity levels create a more comfortable sleeping environment by preventing dry air that can cause skin irritation, dry eyes, and throat irritation. This promotes deeper, more restful sleep and reduces

the likelihood of waking up during the night due to discomfort.

4. **Prevents Dryness**: Dry air can exacerbate symptoms of respiratory infections and allergies, making it harder to recover from illness. Humidifiers help maintain adequate moisture levels in the air, preventing dryness and irritation in the respiratory tract and promoting faster healing.

5. **Reduces Snoring**: Proper humidification can help reduce snoring by keeping the airways moist and reducing inflammation and congestion in the nasal passages and throat. This can lead to quieter and more restful sleep for both the snorer and their sleeping partner.

6. **Enhances Skin Health**: Humidifiers can benefit skin health by preventing dryness and promoting hydration. Properly moisturized air can help maintain the skin's natural moisture barrier, reducing the risk of dry, flaky skin and promoting a healthy complexion.

When using a humidifier in the bedroom, it's essential to follow these tips to ensure safe and effective humidification:

- Choose the Right Type: Select a humidifier that suits your needs and preferences, such as cool mist or warm mist, based on factors like climate, personal comfort, and any specific health concerns.
- Maintain Proper Hygiene: Clean and disinfect your humidifier regularly to prevent the growth of mold, bacteria, and other harmful microorganisms. Follow the manufacturer's instructions for cleaning and maintenance.
- Monitor Humidity Levels: Use a hygrometer to monitor indoor humidity levels and adjust the humidifier settings as needed to maintain optimal humidity levels (ideally between 30-50% relative humidity).
- Position Carefully: Place the humidifier in a safe and stable location away from direct contact with walls or furniture to prevent water damage and ensure proper air circulation.
- Use Distilled Water: Use distilled or demineralized water in your humidifier to prevent mineral buildup and white dust accumulation. This can help maintain the humidifier's efficiency and prolong its lifespan.

By incorporating humidification into your sleep environment, you can create a more comfortable and conducive atmosphere for restful sleep and promote faster recovery from illness.

Using humidifiers is an effective way to relieve congestion and alleviate discomfort associated with respiratory infections such as colds and flu. Here's how humidifiers can help:

1. **Moisturizing the Air**: Humidifiers add moisture to the air, which helps prevent dryness in the nasal passages and throat. Moist air can soothe irritated mucous membranes and reduce inflammation, making it easier to breathe and relieving congestion.

2. **Loosening Mucus**: Increased humidity can help loosen thick mucus and congestion in the respiratory tract. This makes it easier for the body to expel mucus through coughing or blowing the nose, providing relief from congestion and promoting clearer breathing.

3. **Reducing Irritation**: Dry air can irritate the respiratory tract, exacerbating symptoms of congestion, sore throat, and coughing. Humidifiers help maintain optimal humidity levels in the air, preventing dryness and reducing irritation in the nose, throat, and lungs.

4. **Promoting Comfortable Breathing**: Proper humidity levels create a more comfortable breathing environment, especially for individuals with nasal congestion or respiratory conditions. Moist air can help open up nasal passages and airways, allowing for easier and more comfortable breathing.

5. **Improving Sleep Quality**: Congestion can interfere with sleep quality by causing discomfort and difficulty breathing, particularly when lying down. Using a humidifier in the bedroom can help alleviate congestion and promote clearer breathing, leading to better sleep quality and more restful nights.

When using a humidifier to relieve congestion, consider the following tips for optimal effectiveness and safety:

- Choose the Right Type: Select a humidifier that suits your needs and preferences, such as cool mist or warm mist, based on factors like climate, personal comfort, and any specific health concerns.
- Clean Regularly: Clean and disinfect your humidifier regularly to prevent the growth of mold, bacteria, and other harmful microorganisms. Follow the manufacturer's instructions for cleaning

and maintenance to ensure safe and effective operation.
- Use Distilled Water: Use distilled or demineralized water in your humidifier to prevent mineral buildup and white dust accumulation. This can help maintain the humidifier's efficiency and prolong its lifespan.
- Monitor Humidity Levels: Use a hygrometer to monitor indoor humidity levels and adjust the humidifier settings as needed to maintain optimal humidity levels (ideally between 30-50% relative humidity).
- Position Carefully: Place the humidifier in a safe and stable location away from direct contact with walls or furniture to prevent water damage and ensure proper air circulation.

By using a humidifier to relieve congestion, you can create a more comfortable and soothing environment for respiratory health and promote clearer breathing during times of illness.

Natural humidification methods can help increase moisture in the air without the use of electronic devices. Here are some effective natural ways to humidify your home:

1. **Houseplants**:
   - Place indoor plants throughout your home to naturally increase humidity levels. Plants release moisture through a process called transpiration, which can help humidify the air in indoor spaces.
   - Choose moisture-loving plants such as peace lilies, spider plants, ferns, and orchids to maximize humidity levels.

2. **Open Water Containers**:
   - Place shallow bowls or containers filled with water near heat sources such as radiators or heaters. As the water evaporates, it adds moisture to the air, increasing humidity levels in the room.
   - You can also place water-filled trays or bowls on top of or near heating vents to facilitate evaporation and humidification.

3. **Damp Towels or Sheets**:
   - Hang damp towels or sheets near heat sources or in areas with dry air. As the water evaporates from the fabric, it releases moisture into the surrounding air, increasing humidity levels.
   - Be sure to wring out excess water from the towels or sheets to prevent dripping and water damage to surfaces.

4. **Use a Stovetop Potpourri**:
   - Simmer a pot of water on the stove and add aromatic ingredients such as citrus slices, cinnamon sticks, cloves, or herbs like rosemary and thyme.
   - As the water evaporates, it releases moisture and a pleasant aroma into the air, naturally humidifying your home while adding a refreshing scent.

5. **Hang Laundry to Dry Indoors**:
   - Hang wet laundry to dry indoors instead of using a dryer. As the moisture evaporates from the clothes, it increases humidity levels in the room.
   - This method not only humidifies the air but also saves energy by reducing the need for dryer usage.

6. **Use a Room Fountain or Water Feature**:
   - Install a small fountain or water feature in your home to create a natural source of humidity. The movement of water and the sound of flowing water can add a soothing ambiance to your living space while increasing humidity levels.

7. **Ventilation**:
   - Open windows and doors during humid weather to allow moisture from the outside air to enter your home. This can help increase indoor humidity levels

naturally, especially in areas with high outdoor humidity.

By incorporating these natural humidification methods into your home, you can increase moisture levels in the air and create a more comfortable and healthy indoor environment, especially during dry winter months or in arid climates.

Chapter 8

Nutrition and Diet

1. **Importance of Nutrition**:
   - A well-balanced diet plays a crucial role in supporting overall health and immune function, which is essential for preventing and managing colds and flu.

2. **Key Nutrients for Immune Health**:
   - Vitamin C: Found in citrus fruits, bell peppers, strawberries, and leafy greens, vitamin C supports immune function and helps reduce the severity and duration of cold symptoms.
   - Vitamin D: Sunlight exposure, fatty fish, fortified dairy products, and supplements can provide vitamin D, which is important for immune regulation and respiratory health.
   - Zinc: Sources include lean meats, poultry, seafood, nuts, seeds, and whole grains. Zinc helps reduce the duration and severity of cold symptoms and supports immune function.
   - Omega-3 fatty acids: Found in fatty fish, flaxseeds, chia seeds, and walnuts, omega-3 fatty acids have anti-inflammatory properties that can help reduce inflammation in the body and support immune function.

3. **Antioxidant-Rich Foods**:
   - Incorporate antioxidant-rich foods such as berries, nuts, seeds, dark leafy greens, and colorful fruits and vegetables into your diet. Antioxidants help protect cells from damage caused by harmful free radicals and support overall health and immunity.

4. **Hydration**:
   - Drink plenty of fluids, including water, herbal teas, broths, and soups, to stay hydrated and support proper immune function. Adequate hydration helps maintain mucous membrane integrity and supports the body's natural defense mechanisms.

5. **Protein-Rich Foods**:
   - Include lean sources of protein such as poultry, fish, eggs, beans, lentils, tofu, and low-fat dairy products in your diet. Protein is essential for building and repairing tissues, including those involved in immune function.

6. **Garlic and Onions**:
   - Incorporate garlic and onions into your meals, as they contain compounds with antimicrobial and immune-boosting properties. These ingredients can

help support immune function and reduce the risk of infections.

7. **Probiotic Foods**:
   - Consume probiotic-rich foods such as yogurt, kefir, sauerkraut, kimchi, and kombucha to support gut health and immune function. Probiotics help maintain a healthy balance of beneficial bacteria in the gut, which plays a crucial role in immune regulation.

8. **Limit Sugar and Processed Foods**:
   - Minimize consumption of sugary snacks, beverages, and processed foods, as excessive sugar intake can suppress immune function and increase susceptibility to infections. Focus on whole, nutrient-dense foods to support optimal health and immunity.

9. **Moderate Alcohol Intake**:
   - Limit alcohol consumption, as excessive alcohol intake can impair immune function and disrupt sleep patterns, making it harder for the body to fight off infections.

10. **Balanced Meals and Snacks**:
    - Aim for balanced meals and snacks that include a variety of nutrient-rich foods from all food groups

to ensure you're getting essential vitamins, minerals, and antioxidants to support immune health.

By prioritizing a nutrient-rich diet that includes a variety of fruits, vegetables, lean proteins, whole grains, and healthy fats, you can support immune function, promote overall health, and reduce the risk of colds and flu. Additionally, staying hydrated and minimizing consumption of sugary and processed foods can further bolster your body's defenses against illness.

Foods to Eat During Cold and Flu:

1. **Broths and Soups**:
   - Chicken noodle soup, vegetable soup, or bone broth are hydrating and provide essential nutrients to support recovery. The warm liquid can soothe a sore throat and provide comfort.

2. **Citrus Fruits**:
   - Oranges, lemons, grapefruits, and limes are rich in vitamin C, which can help boost the immune system and reduce the severity of cold symptoms.

3. **Berries**:
   - Blueberries, strawberries, raspberries, and blackberries are packed with antioxidants that help fight off infections and reduce inflammation.

4. **Garlic and Onions**:
   - Garlic and onions contain compounds with antimicrobial properties that can help combat cold and flu viruses. Incorporate them into soups, stews, and stir-fries for added flavor and health benefits.

5. **Ginger**:
   - Ginger has anti-inflammatory and soothing properties that can help relieve nausea, sore throat, and congestion. Enjoy ginger tea or add fresh ginger to soups and smoothies.

6. **Honey**:
   - Honey has antimicrobial properties and can help soothe a sore throat and cough. Add honey to herbal teas or consume it plain for relief.

7. **Yogurt and Probiotic Foods**:
   - Yogurt, kefir, sauerkraut, and kimchi contain probiotics that support gut health and immune function. Choose unsweetened yogurt for the best health benefits.

8. **Turmeric**:
   - Turmeric contains curcumin, a compound with anti-inflammatory and antioxidant properties. Add turmeric to soups, curries, or golden milk for its immune-boosting benefits.

9. **Leafy Greens**:
   - Spinach, kale, Swiss chard, and other leafy greens are rich in vitamins, minerals, and antioxidants that support immune function and overall health.

10. **Oily Fish**:
    - Salmon, mackerel, and sardines are high in omega-3 fatty acids, which have anti-inflammatory properties that can help reduce inflammation and support immune health.

11. **Hot Tea with Lemon and Honey**:
    - Herbal teas such as chamomile, peppermint, and echinacea can provide hydration and soothing relief for cold symptoms. Add lemon for vitamin C and honey for its antimicrobial properties.

12. **Whole Grains**:
    - Whole grains like oats, brown rice, quinoa, and barley provide energy and essential nutrients to support the body's immune response during illness.

13. **Poultry**:
   - Chicken and turkey contain protein and essential amino acids that support immune function and promote recovery. Enjoy lean cuts of poultry in soups, salads, or sandwiches.

14. **Spicy Foods**:
   - Spicy foods like chili peppers, horseradish, and mustard can help clear nasal congestion and stimulate the release of mucus, providing relief from cold symptoms.

15. **Fluids**:
   - Stay hydrated by drinking plenty of water, herbal teas, broths, and electrolyte-rich beverages like coconut water to support hydration and recovery.

Incorporating these nutrient-rich foods into your diet during cold and flu can help support immune function, reduce inflammation, and alleviate symptoms, promoting faster recovery and overall well-being.

Foods to Avoid During Cold and Flu:

1. **Sugary Foods and Beverages**:

- Avoid sugary snacks, candies, sodas, and sweetened beverages as they can suppress immune function and worsen inflammation.

2. **Processed Foods**:
   - Limit consumption of processed and packaged foods high in refined carbohydrates, unhealthy fats, and artificial additives. These foods offer little nutritional value and can weaken the immune system.

3. **Fried and Greasy Foods**:
   - Steer clear of fried foods, fast food, and greasy snacks, as they can be difficult to digest and may exacerbate gastrointestinal symptoms such as nausea or indigestion.

4. **Alcohol**:
   - Avoid alcohol, as it can dehydrate the body, impair immune function, and disrupt sleep patterns, which are essential for recovery from illness.

5. **Caffeinated Beverages**:
   - Limit consumption of caffeinated beverages such as coffee, black tea, and energy drinks, as they can interfere with hydration and disrupt sleep, leading to fatigue and impaired immune function.

6. **Dairy Products (for Some Individuals)**:
   - Some people may find that dairy products exacerbate congestion and mucus production during colds and flu. If you experience increased mucus or congestion after consuming dairy, consider reducing or avoiding dairy products temporarily.

7. **Spicy and Acidic Foods**:
   - Spicy foods, acidic foods, and condiments like hot sauce, vinegar, and citrus may irritate a sore throat or exacerbate gastrointestinal symptoms, so it's best to avoid them if you're feeling unwell.

8. **Excessive Salt**:
   - Minimize consumption of highly salty foods such as chips, processed snacks, and canned soups, as excessive salt intake can contribute to dehydration and exacerbate inflammation.

9. **Large Meals**:
   - Avoid consuming large, heavy meals that can put a strain on digestion and energy levels. Opt for smaller, lighter meals and snacks that are easier to digest and provide steady energy throughout the day.

10. **Raw or Undercooked Foods**:
   - During illness, it's best to avoid raw or undercooked foods, including meats, seafood, eggs, and unpasteurized dairy products, to reduce the risk of foodborne illness and gastrointestinal upset.

11. **Excessive Spices and Seasonings**:
   - While herbs and spices can add flavor and nutrients to meals, excessive use of strong spices and seasonings may irritate the digestive tract or exacerbate symptoms of nausea or indigestion.

12. **Cigarettes and Tobacco Products**:
   - If you smoke, avoid cigarettes and tobacco products during colds and flu, as smoking can worsen respiratory symptoms, impair immune function, and delay recovery from illness.

By avoiding these foods and beverages during colds and flu, you can support immune function, reduce inflammation, and alleviate symptoms, promoting faster recovery and overall well-being. Instead, focus on consuming nutrient-rich foods and staying hydrated to support your body's natural healing processes.

Chapter 9

Alternative Therapies

Alternative therapies can complement conventional treatments and help alleviate symptoms of colds and flu. Here are some alternative therapies to consider:

1. **Acupuncture**:
   - Acupuncture involves the insertion of thin needles into specific points on the body to stimulate energy flow and promote healing. It may help alleviate symptoms such as congestion, headache, and body aches associated with colds and flu.

2. **Herbal Medicine**:
   - Herbal remedies, including teas, tinctures, and supplements, can support immune function and help relieve symptoms of colds and flu. Popular herbs for colds and flu include echinacea, elderberry, ginger, and licorice root.

3. **Homeopathy**:
   - Homeopathic remedies use highly diluted substances to stimulate the body's natural healing processes. Remedies such as Oscillococcinum and

Arsenicum album are commonly used for colds and flu symptoms.

4. **Aromatherapy**:
   - Aromatherapy involves the use of essential oils to promote physical and emotional well-being. Inhalation, massage, and diffusion of oils such as eucalyptus, peppermint, lavender, and tea tree can help relieve congestion, ease muscle tension, and support relaxation during illness.

5. **Naturopathy**:
   - Naturopathic medicine focuses on holistic approaches to health, including nutrition, lifestyle modifications, and natural therapies. Naturopathic doctors may recommend dietary changes, supplements, hydrotherapy, and other natural treatments to support immune function and alleviate symptoms of colds and flu.

6. **Chiropractic Care**:
   - Chiropractic adjustments can help improve spinal alignment and nervous system function, which may support immune function and overall health. Some people find relief from cold and flu symptoms through chiropractic adjustments.

7. **Traditional Chinese Medicine (TCM)**:
   - TCM includes modalities such as acupuncture, herbal medicine, cupping, and qigong to restore balance and harmony in the body. TCM practitioners may prescribe customized herbal formulas and acupuncture treatments to address cold and flu symptoms based on individual patterns of imbalance.

8. **Massage Therapy**:
   - Massage therapy can help reduce muscle tension, improve circulation, and promote relaxation during illness. Gentle massage techniques, such as Swedish massage or lymphatic drainage massage, may help ease symptoms and support the body's natural healing processes.

9. **Hydrotherapy**:
   - Hydrotherapy involves the use of water in various forms (such as hot baths, steam baths, and contrast showers) to promote relaxation, stimulate circulation, and support detoxification. Hydrotherapy can help relieve congestion, soothe sore muscles, and promote overall well-being during colds and flu.

10. **Mind-Body Practices**:
   - Mind-body practices such as yoga, tai chi, meditation, and deep breathing exercises can help reduce stress, support immune function, and promote relaxation during illness. These practices may also enhance overall resilience and well-being.

When considering alternative therapies for colds and flu, it's essential to consult with qualified practitioners and inform your healthcare provider about any complementary treatments you're considering. Integrating alternative therapies with conventional treatments can provide a holistic approach to managing symptoms and promoting recovery from colds and flu.

Acupuncture is an ancient healing practice rooted in traditional Chinese medicine (TCM) that involves the insertion of thin needles into specific points on the body to balance the flow of energy, or qi (pronounced "chee"), along meridian pathways. Here's how acupuncture works to balance energy flow:

1. **Meridian System**:
   - According to TCM theory, the body contains a network of meridians, or energy channels, through

which qi flows. There are 12 main meridians, each associated with specific organs and bodily functions.

2. **Qi and Health**:
   - Qi is believed to be the vital life force that animates the body and maintains health and vitality. When qi becomes blocked or imbalanced, it can lead to pain, illness, and dysfunction.

3. **Acupuncture Points**:
   - Acupuncture points are specific locations along the meridians where qi can be accessed and manipulated. These points are thought to correspond to various organs, tissues, and functions of the body.

4. **Needle Stimulation**:
   - Acupuncture involves the insertion of thin, sterile needles into acupuncture points to stimulate and regulate the flow of qi. The needles are typically inserted to varying depths depending on the individual's condition and the desired therapeutic effect.

5. **Balancing Qi**:
   - Acupuncture aims to restore balance and harmony within the body by regulating the flow of

qi. Depending on the individual's presentation, acupuncture may tonify deficient qi, disperse excess qi, or harmonize imbalances between yin and yang energies.

6. **Effects on the Body**:
   - Acupuncture can have a variety of physiological effects on the body, including:
   - Stimulating the release of endorphins and other neurotransmitters, which can help reduce pain and promote relaxation.
   - Modulating the activity of the autonomic nervous system, which regulates functions such as heart rate, digestion, and immune response.
   - Increasing blood flow and circulation to promote healing and tissue repair.
   - Regulating inflammatory and immune responses to support overall health and well-being.

7. **Holistic Approach**:
   - Acupuncture is often used as part of a comprehensive treatment plan that may include dietary modifications, herbal remedies, lifestyle changes, and other complementary therapies. By addressing imbalances in the body's energy system, acupuncture aims to promote optimal health and vitality on physical, emotional, and spiritual levels.

Overall, acupuncture is based on the principle of restoring balance and harmony within the body's energy system to support health and well-being. Through the gentle stimulation of acupuncture points, acupuncture can help regulate the flow of qi and alleviate a wide range of symptoms and conditions, including those associated with colds and flu.

Homeopathy is a holistic system of medicine that uses highly diluted substances to stimulate the body's natural healing processes. Central to homeopathy is the principle of "like cures like," which means that a substance that causes symptoms in a healthy person can be used to treat similar symptoms in someone who is unwell. Here's how homeopathy provides individualized treatment for symptoms:

1. **Patient-Centered Approach**:
   - Homeopathy takes into account the unique symptoms, characteristics, and experiences of each individual patient. Homeopaths conduct thorough interviews and assessments to understand the physical, mental, and emotional aspects of a person's health.

2. **Symptom Matching**:
   - Homeopathic remedies are selected based on the principle of symptom similarity. The homeopath evaluates the totality of symptoms experienced by the patient and selects a remedy that closely matches the person's unique symptom profile.

3. **Individualization of Treatment**:
   - Homeopathic treatment is highly individualized, with different remedies chosen for different patients based on their specific symptoms, constitution, and overall health status. What works for one person may not work for another, even if they have similar symptoms.

4. **Potentization**:
   - Homeopathic remedies are prepared through a process called potentization, which involves serial dilution and succussion (vigorous shaking). This process removes the original substance's material properties while retaining its energetic essence or healing potential.

5. **Minimum Dose**:
   - Homeopathic remedies are administered in highly diluted and potentized forms, often in the form of sugar pellets or liquid tinctures. The use of minimal doses reduces the risk of toxicity and side

effects while maximizing the remedy's therapeutic effects.

6. **Dynamic Medicine**:
   - Homeopathic remedies work on an energetic level to stimulate the body's vital force or innate healing capacity. Rather than suppressing symptoms, homeopathy aims to support the body's self-healing mechanisms and restore balance and harmony.

7. **Self-Healing Response**:
   - Homeopathic remedies are believed to stimulate the body's self-healing response, triggering a cascade of physiological and biochemical changes that promote healing and resolution of symptoms.

8. **Complementary and Integrative Care**:
   - Homeopathy can be used alone or as part of a comprehensive treatment plan that may include conventional medicine, lifestyle modifications, dietary changes, and other complementary therapies. Homeopaths often work collaboratively with other healthcare providers to optimize patient care.

Overall, homeopathy provides individualized treatment for symptoms by matching specific remedies to the unique symptom profile of each patient. By addressing the underlying causes of illness and supporting the body's innate healing mechanisms, homeopathy aims to promote holistic health and well-being.

Chapter 10

Exercise and Movement

Exercise and movement play crucial roles in maintaining overall health and supporting immune function, which can help prevent and alleviate symptoms of colds and flu. Here's how exercise and movement contribute to health during colds and flu:

1. **Boosting Immune Function**:
   - Regular exercise has been shown to enhance immune function by increasing circulation, promoting the production of immune cells, and reducing inflammation. This can help strengthen the body's defenses against colds, flu, and other infections.

2. **Reducing Stress**:
   - Exercise helps reduce stress levels by releasing endorphins, neurotransmitters that promote feelings of well-being and relaxation. Managing stress is essential for maintaining a healthy immune system and reducing susceptibility to illness.

3. **Improving Respiratory Health**:
   - Moderate aerobic exercise, such as brisk walking, cycling, or swimming, can improve respiratory function and lung capacity. This may help alleviate symptoms of congestion and promote clearer breathing during colds and flu.

4. **Enhancing Circulation**:
   - Physical activity increases blood flow and circulation throughout the body, delivering oxygen and nutrients to tissues and organs. Improved circulation can support the body's natural healing processes and aid in recovery from illness.

5. **Promoting Detoxification**:
   - Sweating during exercise helps eliminate toxins from the body through the skin. This can support detoxification and elimination of waste products, potentially reducing the duration and severity of illness.

6. **Maintaining Healthy Weight**:
   - Regular exercise helps maintain a healthy weight and body composition, which is important for overall health and immune function. Excess body weight can increase the risk of chronic diseases and impair immune responses.

7. **Enhancing Mood and Mental Health**:
   - Exercise has mood-boosting effects and can help alleviate symptoms of depression, anxiety, and stress. Maintaining positive mental health is important for overall well-being and immune function.

8. **Improving Sleep Quality**:
   - Regular physical activity can improve sleep quality and duration, which is essential for immune function and recovery from illness. Adequate restorative sleep supports immune responses and enhances the body's ability to fight off infections.

9. **Promoting Lymphatic Drainage**:
   - Movement and exercise help stimulate lymphatic circulation, facilitating the removal of waste products, toxins, and pathogens from the body. This can support immune function and reduce the risk of infection.

10. **Moderation and Rest During Illness**:
    - While regular exercise is beneficial for overall health, it's important to listen to your body and rest when you're feeling unwell. During colds and flu, prioritize gentle movement such as stretching, yoga, or short walks, and avoid intense or strenuous exercise until you've fully recovered.

Incorporating regular exercise and movement into your daily routine can support immune function, promote overall health, and reduce the risk of colds and flu. Additionally, staying active during illness, while also prioritizing rest and recovery, can help alleviate symptoms and support the body's natural healing processes.

Gentle exercise can be beneficial for symptom relief during colds and flu, as it helps promote circulation, reduce muscle tension, and support overall well-being without placing undue stress on the body. Here are some gentle exercises and movement practices that may provide relief:

1. **Walking**:
   - Taking short, leisurely walks can help increase circulation, clear the mind, and improve mood during illness. Aim for a gentle pace and listen to your body's cues to avoid overexertion.

2. **Yoga**:
   - Gentle yoga poses and stretches can help relieve muscle tension, improve flexibility, and promote relaxation. Choose restorative or yin yoga practices that focus on gentle stretching, deep breathing, and mindfulness.

3. **Tai Chi**:
   - Tai Chi is a gentle form of movement that involves slow, flowing movements and deep breathing. It can help improve balance, coordination, and relaxation while promoting a sense of calm and well-being.

4. **Qi Gong**:
   - Qi Gong combines gentle movements, breathwork, and meditation to promote energy flow and balance within the body. It can help reduce stress, enhance vitality, and support immune function during illness.

5. **Pilates**:
   - Pilates focuses on core strength, flexibility, and body awareness through controlled movements and breathwork. Choose gentle Pilates exercises that emphasize alignment and low-impact movements to support recovery from illness.

6. **Stretching**:
   - Gentle stretching exercises can help relieve muscle stiffness and tension, improve flexibility, and promote relaxation. Focus on slow, controlled stretches that target areas of tightness or discomfort.

7. **Breathing Exercises**:
   - Practicing deep breathing exercises can help reduce stress, promote relaxation, and support respiratory function during illness. Try diaphragmatic breathing, alternate nostril breathing, or guided relaxation techniques to calm the mind and body.

8. **Swimming or Water Aerobics**:
   - If you're feeling up to it, gentle swimming or water aerobics in a warm pool can provide soothing relief for sore muscles and joints while promoting gentle movement and relaxation.

9. **Gentle Stretching**:
   - Perform gentle stretching exercises targeting areas of tension, such as neck stretches, shoulder rolls, and gentle twists. Hold each stretch for 15-30 seconds and avoid bouncing or overstretching.

10. **Mindful Movement**:
    - Engage in activities that promote mindfulness and present-moment awareness, such as walking meditation, mindful stretching, or gentle movement practices like Feldenkrais or Alexander Technique.

When engaging in gentle exercise during colds and flu, listen to your body's signals and avoid pushing yourself too hard. Rest as needed, stay hydrated, and prioritize self-care to support your body's natural healing processes. If you experience severe symptoms or worsening of illness, consult with a healthcare professional before resuming exercise.

Yoga and stretching are excellent practices for promoting relaxation, reducing stress, and relieving tension in the body and mind. Here's how you can incorporate yoga and stretching into your routine for relaxation during colds and flu:

1. **Gentle Yoga Poses**:
   - Choose gentle yoga poses that focus on deep breathing, gentle stretching, and relaxation. Poses such as Child's Pose (Balasana), Cat-Cow Stretch, and Legs-Up-The-Wall Pose (Viparita Karani) can help release tension and promote relaxation.

2. **Deep Breathing Techniques**:
   - Practice deep breathing exercises, such as diaphragmatic breathing (also known as belly breathing), to calm the nervous system and induce a state of relaxation. Combine deep breathing with gentle yoga poses for added relaxation benefits.

3. **Restorative Yoga**:
   - Restorative yoga involves passive, supported poses held for extended periods to promote deep relaxation and stress relief. Use props such as blankets, bolsters, and pillows to support your body in gentle, restful poses like Supported Bridge Pose or Reclining Bound Angle Pose.

4. **Seated Forward Fold (Paschimottanasana)**:
   - Sit on the floor with your legs extended in front of you. Slowly fold forward from the hips, reaching your hands toward your feet or resting them on your legs. Keep your spine long and your breath deep as you gently stretch the back of your body. Hold the pose for several breaths, then slowly release.

5. **Neck and Shoulder Stretches**:
   - Gently stretch the neck and shoulders to relieve tension and promote relaxation. Try gentle neck rolls, shoulder shrugs, and side neck stretches to release tightness in the upper body.

6. **Supine Twist**:
   - Lie on your back with your knees bent and feet flat on the floor. Extend your arms out to the sides in a T-position. Slowly lower both knees to one side,

keeping your shoulders grounded. Hold the twist for a few breaths, then switch sides. This pose helps release tension in the spine and promotes relaxation.

7. **Savasana (Corpse Pose)**:
   - End your yoga or stretching session with Savasana, a pose of total relaxation. Lie on your back with your legs extended and arms by your sides, palms facing up. Close your eyes and allow your body to relax completely, focusing on your breath and letting go of tension with each exhale.

8. **Guided Relaxation or Meditation**:
   - Incorporate guided relaxation or meditation practices into your yoga or stretching routine to enhance relaxation and promote mental calmness. Use gentle imagery, soothing music, or guided meditation recordings to guide you into a state of deep relaxation.

By incorporating yoga and stretching practices into your routine, you can promote relaxation, reduce stress, and relieve tension in the body and mind, supporting your overall well-being during colds and flu. Remember to listen to your body and modify poses as needed to suit your comfort level and current health condition.

Chapter 11

Home Remedies for Children

Home remedies for children can provide gentle relief from symptoms of colds and flu while supporting their immune system and overall well-being. Here are some effective and safe home remedies for children:

1. **Plenty of Rest**:
   - Ensure your child gets plenty of rest to support their body's natural healing processes. Encourage quiet activities such as reading, coloring, or watching movies to help them relax and recuperate.

2. **Hydration**:
   - Keep your child well-hydrated by offering plenty of fluids such as water, herbal teas, diluted fruit juices, and clear broths. Staying hydrated helps soothe sore throats, thin mucus, and prevent dehydration.

3. **Warm Liquids**:
   - Offer warm liquids such as herbal teas, warm water with honey, or chicken broth to help soothe sore throats, relieve congestion, and provide comfort.

4. **Humidifier**:
   - Use a cool-mist humidifier in your child's room to add moisture to the air and help ease congestion and coughing. Clean the humidifier regularly to prevent the growth of mold and bacteria.

5. **Nasal Saline Drops**:
   - Use saline nasal drops or spray to help loosen nasal congestion and clear mucus from your child's nasal passages. Saline drops are safe and gentle for children of all ages.

6. **Steam Therapy**:
   - Create a steamy environment in the bathroom by running a hot shower or bath and sitting with your child in the steam-filled room for a few minutes. Steam helps loosen congestion and ease breathing.

7. **Honey**:
   - For children over one year of age, honey can help soothe coughs and sore throats. Offer a teaspoon of honey alone or mix it with warm water or herbal tea. Never give honey to children under one year of age due to the risk of infant botulism.

8. **Warm Salt Gargle**:
   - For older children who can safely gargle, a warm saltwater gargle can help soothe sore throats and

reduce inflammation. Mix a teaspoon of salt in warm water and have your child gargle with the solution for a few seconds before spitting it out.

9. **Chicken Soup**:
   - Warm chicken soup can provide nourishment, hydration, and comfort to children with colds and flu. Homemade chicken soup with vegetables contains nutrients that support immune function and promote healing.

10. **Proper Nutrition**:
    - Offer your child a balanced diet rich in fruits, vegetables, whole grains, and lean proteins to support their immune system and overall health. Limit sugary snacks and processed foods that can weaken immunity.

11. **Encourage Nasal Blowing**:
    - Teach your child how to blow their nose gently to help clear congestion and alleviate discomfort. Provide soft tissues or wipes to prevent irritation of the skin around the nose.

12. **Warm Compresses**:
    - Apply a warm, moist washcloth to your child's forehead, sinuses, or chest to help relieve

congestion, ease muscle tension, and provide comfort.

Always consult with your child's pediatrician before administering any home remedies, especially if your child has underlying health conditions or is taking medication. Additionally, monitor your child's symptoms closely and seek medical attention if they worsen or persist for an extended period.

Safe and effective remedies for kids can help alleviate symptoms of colds and flu while supporting their immune system and overall well-being. Here are some recommended remedies:

1. **Hydration**:
   - Encourage your child to drink plenty of fluids such as water, herbal teas, diluted fruit juices, and clear broths to stay hydrated and help loosen mucus.

2. **Rest**:
   - Ensure your child gets plenty of rest to support their body's healing process. Allow them to stay home from school or daycare to rest and recover fully.

3. **Nasal Saline Drops**:
   - Use saline nasal drops or spray to help relieve nasal congestion and clear mucus from your child's nasal passages. Saline drops are safe and gentle for children of all ages.

4. **Humidifier**:
   - Use a cool-mist humidifier in your child's room to add moisture to the air and help ease congestion, coughing, and sore throat. Clean the humidifier regularly to prevent mold and bacteria growth.

5. **Warm Liquids**:
   - Offer warm liquids such as herbal teas, warm water with honey, or chicken broth to soothe sore throats, ease coughing, and provide comfort.

6. **Honey**:
   - For children over one year of age, honey can help relieve coughs and soothe sore throats. Offer a teaspoon of honey alone or mix it with warm water or herbal tea. Do not give honey to children under one year of age due to the risk of infant botulism.

7. **Chicken Soup**:
   - Warm chicken soup can provide nourishment, hydration, and comfort to children with colds and flu. Homemade chicken soup with vegetables

contains nutrients that support immune function and promote healing.

8. **Proper Nutrition**:
   - Offer your child a balanced diet rich in fruits, vegetables, whole grains, and lean proteins to support their immune system and overall health. Limit sugary snacks and processed foods that can weaken immunity.

9. **Frequent Handwashing**:
   - Encourage your child to wash their hands frequently with soap and water to prevent the spread of germs and reduce the risk of infection.

10. **Warm Baths**:
    - A warm bath can help relax your child's muscles, relieve congestion, and provide soothing comfort. Add a few drops of eucalyptus or lavender essential oil to the bathwater for additional respiratory support and relaxation.

11. **Elevating the Head**:
    - Elevate your child's head while sleeping to help ease congestion and promote better breathing. Use extra pillows or raise the head of the bed slightly to achieve a comfortable elevation.

12. **Over-the-Counter Medications**:
   - Use over-the-counter medications such as children's acetaminophen or ibuprofen to reduce fever and relieve pain if recommended by your child's pediatrician. Follow dosing instructions carefully based on your child's age and weight.

Always consult with your child's pediatrician before administering any home remedies or over-the-counter medications, especially if your child has underlying health conditions or is taking medication. Additionally, monitor your child's symptoms closely and seek medical attention if they worsen or persist for an extended period.

Dosage and precautions for administering remedies to children are essential to ensure their safety and effectiveness. Here are some general guidelines:

1. **Dosage**:
   - Always follow the recommended dosage instructions provided on the product packaging or as directed by your child's healthcare provider. Dosages may vary based on your child's age, weight, and specific health condition.

2. **Age Appropriateness**:
   - Check the age recommendations for each remedy to ensure it is suitable for your child's age group. Some remedies may not be safe for infants or young children, while others may have specific formulations for different age ranges.

3. **Weight Consideration**:
   - Pay attention to dosage recommendations based on your child's weight, especially for medications and supplements. Use a pediatric dosing chart or consult with your child's healthcare provider if you are unsure about the appropriate dosage.

4. **Administration**:
   - Administer remedies in the appropriate form and method as directed. For example, some medications may need to be administered with food to reduce stomach upset, while others may need to be diluted in water or juice for easier ingestion.

5. **Frequency**:
   - Follow the recommended dosing frequency for each remedy. Avoid giving medications or supplements more frequently than recommended unless advised by your child's healthcare provider.

6. **Precautions**:
   - Be aware of any potential side effects or contraindications associated with the remedies you are using. Monitor your child closely for any adverse reactions and discontinue use if necessary.

7. **Allergies and Sensitivities**:
   - Be mindful of any allergies or sensitivities your child may have to ingredients in remedies. Check the product labels for allergen information and consult with your child's healthcare provider if you have concerns.

8. **Interaction with Medications**:
   - If your child is taking any prescription medications, consult with their healthcare provider before administering any over-the-counter remedies or supplements to avoid potential interactions.

9. **Storage**:
   - Store remedies safely out of reach of children and in accordance with the manufacturer's instructions. Keep medications and supplements in their original packaging and away from heat, moisture, and direct sunlight.

10. **Seek Medical Advice**:
   - If you have any questions or concerns about dosage, administration, or safety precautions, consult with your child's healthcare provider before giving any remedies. They can provide personalized guidance based on your child's individual needs and health status.

By following proper dosage and precautions, you can ensure the safe and effective use of remedies for your child's colds and flu symptoms. Always prioritize your child's safety and well-being, and seek medical advice if you have any doubts or concerns.

Chapter 12

When to Seek Medical Attention

It's important to monitor your child's symptoms closely and seek medical attention if any of the following occur:

1. **High Fever**:
   - If your child has a fever of 100.4°F (38°C) or higher, especially if they are under three months of age, seek medical advice. Persistent or high fever can indicate a more serious infection that may require medical attention.

2. **Difficulty Breathing**:
   - If your child is experiencing difficulty breathing, rapid breathing, or wheezing, seek immediate medical attention. These symptoms may indicate respiratory distress or infection that requires prompt evaluation and treatment.

3. **Severe or Persistent Symptoms**:
   - If your child's symptoms are severe, worsening, or persisting for more than a few days, consult with their healthcare provider. This includes symptoms such as severe coughing, chest pain, persistent vomiting, or extreme fatigue.

4. **Dehydration**:
   - Watch for signs of dehydration, including decreased urine output, dry mouth, sunken eyes, lethargy, or extreme thirst. If you suspect your child is dehydrated, seek medical attention promptly, especially if they are unable to tolerate fluids or are experiencing diarrhea or vomiting.

5. **Severe Pain or Discomfort**:
   - If your child is experiencing severe pain, discomfort, or distress, seek medical advice. This may include severe headache, ear pain, abdominal pain, or any other localized pain that is causing significant discomfort.

6. **Persistent High-Risk Symptoms**:
   - If your child has underlying health conditions such as asthma, diabetes, or immune disorders, or if they are at higher risk for complications due to their age (e.g., infants, elderly), consult with their healthcare provider for guidance on managing their symptoms and when to seek medical attention.

7. **Unusual Symptoms**:
   - If your child develops unusual symptoms or reactions to remedies or medications, such as rash, swelling, dizziness, or behavioral changes, stop the treatment and seek medical advice.

8. **Concerns or Questions**:
   - If you have any concerns or questions about your child's condition, symptoms, or treatment, don't hesitate to contact their healthcare provider for guidance and advice. Trust your instincts as a parent and seek medical attention if you feel that your child's condition warrants it.

It's always better to err on the side of caution and seek medical attention if you're unsure about your child's symptoms or if you have any concerns about their health and well-being. Your child's healthcare provider can provide personalized guidance and recommendations based on their individual needs and circumstances.

Signs of complications during a cold or flu that may require medical attention include:

1. **High Fever**:
   - A persistent fever of 100.4°F (38°C) or higher, especially in infants under three months old, warrants medical attention. High fever can indicate a more serious infection or complication.

2. **Difficulty Breathing**:
   - Difficulty breathing, rapid or shallow breathing, wheezing, or chest pain while breathing may indicate respiratory complications such as pneumonia or bronchitis.

3. **Persistent Cough**:
   - A cough that persists for more than two weeks or worsens over time, especially if it produces thick, yellow or green mucus, may indicate a respiratory infection or complication.

4. **Severe Headache**:
   - Intense or persistent headache, especially if accompanied by fever, stiff neck, sensitivity to light, confusion, or changes in mental status, may indicate meningitis or another serious condition.

5. **Severe Sore Throat**:
   - Severe throat pain, difficulty swallowing, or the inability to open the mouth fully may indicate tonsillitis, strep throat, or another bacterial infection requiring medical evaluation.

6. **Ear Pain**:
   - Persistent ear pain, especially accompanied by fever, drainage from the ear, or changes in hearing,

may indicate an ear infection that requires medical treatment.

7. **Chest Pain**:
   - Chest pain or discomfort, especially if it worsens with deep breathing or coughing, may indicate inflammation of the chest wall (costochondritis), pleurisy, or other lung complications.

8. **Dehydration**:
   - Signs of dehydration, such as dry mouth, decreased urine output, sunken eyes, lethargy, or extreme thirst, may occur if your child is unable to drink enough fluids due to illness.

9. **Worsening Symptoms**:
   - Any symptoms that worsen over time or fail to improve with home remedies, such as persistent fever, cough, fatigue, or weakness, may indicate a need for medical evaluation.

10. **Decreased Activity Level**:
    - A significant decrease in your child's activity level, energy, or responsiveness, especially if accompanied by other concerning symptoms, may indicate a more serious illness or complication.

11. **Seizures**:
   - Seizures, convulsions, or loss of consciousness may occur in severe cases of flu or other infections and require immediate medical attention.

If you notice any of these signs of complications or have concerns about your child's health, it's important to seek medical attention promptly. Your child's healthcare provider can evaluate their symptoms, provide appropriate treatment, and help prevent further complications.

Consulting a healthcare professional is essential if you observe any of the following concerning signs or if you have any doubts or questions about your child's health during a cold or flu:

1. **Persistent High Fever**:
   - If your child has a fever of 100.4°F (38°C) or higher that persists for more than a few days, especially if they are under three months old, consult their healthcare provider for guidance.

2. **Difficulty Breathing**:
   - If your child experiences difficulty breathing, rapid breathing, wheezing, or chest pain while

breathing, seek medical attention promptly as it may indicate respiratory complications.

3. **Severe Symptoms**:
   - If your child experiences severe symptoms such as severe headache, persistent vomiting, chest pain, or confusion, consult a healthcare professional for evaluation and treatment.

4. **Dehydration**:
   - Signs of dehydration such as dry mouth, decreased urine output, sunken eyes, lethargy, or extreme thirst require medical evaluation and may necessitate intravenous fluids.

5. **Worsening Symptoms**:
   - If your child's symptoms worsen or fail to improve with home remedies, or if they develop new or unusual symptoms, consult their healthcare provider for assessment and appropriate management.

6. **Underlying Health Conditions**:
   - If your child has underlying health conditions such as asthma, diabetes, or immune disorders, or if they are at higher risk for complications due to their age or medical history, consult their

healthcare provider for personalized guidance and management.

7. **Concerns or Questions**:
   - If you have any concerns, questions, or uncertainties about your child's health, symptoms, or treatment, don't hesitate to reach out to their healthcare provider for advice and reassurance.

8. **Medication or Supplement Interactions**:
   - If your child is taking any prescription medications or supplements, consult their healthcare provider before administering any over-the-counter remedies to avoid potential interactions or adverse effects.

9. **Preventive Measures**:
   - Consulting a healthcare professional can also be beneficial for guidance on preventive measures such as vaccination, proper hand hygiene, and lifestyle recommendations to reduce the risk of colds and flu.

10. **Follow-Up Care**:
    - Follow up with your child's healthcare provider as recommended, especially if their symptoms persist or if they experience recurrent infections or complications.

By consulting a healthcare professional, you can receive expert guidance, reassurance, and appropriate management for your child's health concerns, ensuring their well-being and prompt recovery from colds and flu.

Conclusion

In conclusion, colds and flu are common viral infections that can affect children, causing symptoms such as fever, cough, congestion, and sore throat. While these illnesses are usually mild and self-limiting, they can sometimes lead to complications, especially in young children or those with underlying health conditions. However, with proper care and management, most children can recover fully from colds and flu without complications.

Natural home remedies can provide safe and effective relief from symptoms, support immune function, and promote overall well-being in children. From hydration and rest to herbal remedies, steam therapy, and gentle exercises, there are various strategies parents can use to alleviate discomfort and help their child recover more quickly.

It's essential for parents to be vigilant for signs of complications and to seek medical attention if their child's symptoms worsen or if they have concerns about their health. Consulting a healthcare professional can provide reassurance, guidance, and appropriate treatment to ensure the best possible outcome for the child.

By following preventive measures, promoting good hygiene practices, and providing supportive care, parents can help protect their children from colds and flu while supporting their health and well-being throughout the year. With proper attention and care, children can bounce back from illness and continue to thrive.

Here's a recap of the key points regarding managing colds and flu in children:

1. **Understanding Colds and Flu**:
   - Colds and flu are common viral infections in children characterized by symptoms such as fever, cough, congestion, and sore throat.

2. **Importance of Natural Home Remedies**:
   - Natural home remedies can provide safe and effective relief from symptoms, support immune function, and promote overall well-being in children.

3. **Preventive Measures**:
   - Preventive measures such as proper hand hygiene, vaccination, and healthy lifestyle habits can help reduce the risk of colds and flu in children.

4. **Hydration and Rest**:
   - Ensuring adequate hydration and rest is essential for supporting the body's natural healing processes and promoting recovery from illness.

5. **Herbal Remedies and Supplements**:
   - Herbal remedies and supplements such as honey, echinacea, vitamin C, and zinc can help alleviate symptoms and support immune function in children.

6. **Hygiene Practices**:
   - Practicing good hygiene habits such as frequent handwashing, covering coughs and sneezes, and avoiding close contact with sick individuals can help prevent the spread of colds and flu.

7. **Consulting a Healthcare Professional**:
   - Parents should consult a healthcare professional if their child's symptoms worsen, persist, or if they have concerns about their health. Prompt medical attention may be necessary in cases of severe symptoms or complications.

8. **Monitoring for Complications**:
   - Parents should monitor their child closely for signs of complications such as high fever, difficulty breathing, severe headache, or dehydration, and seek medical attention if necessary.

9. **Follow-Up Care**:
   - Follow-up care with a healthcare professional may be necessary, especially if symptoms persist or if the child has underlying health conditions.

10. **Promoting Overall Well-Being**:
    - Supporting a child's overall well-being through healthy nutrition, adequate sleep, regular exercise, and emotional support can help strengthen their immune system and resilience against illness.

By being aware of these key points and implementing appropriate strategies, parents can effectively manage colds and flu in children and promote their health and well-being throughout the year.

Empowering self-care practices for cold and flu can help individuals take charge of their health and well-being while managing symptoms and promoting recovery. Here are some self-care practices for cold and flu:

1. **Stay Hydrated**:
   - Drink plenty of fluids such as water, herbal teas, clear broths, and electrolyte-rich drinks to stay hydrated and help loosen mucus.

2. **Rest and Sleep**:
   - Get plenty of rest and sleep to support the body's natural healing processes and conserve energy for fighting off infection.

3. **Nutritious Diet**:
   - Eat a balanced diet rich in fruits, vegetables, whole grains, and lean proteins to provide essential nutrients that support immune function and overall health.

4. **Herbal Remedies**:
   - Use herbal remedies such as honey, ginger, garlic, and echinacea to help alleviate symptoms and support immune function.

5. **Warm Liquids**:
   - Drink warm liquids such as herbal teas, warm water with honey and lemon, or chicken broth to

soothe sore throat, ease congestion, and provide comfort.

6. **Steam Therapy**:
   - Use steam therapy by inhaling steam from a hot shower or bowl of hot water with essential oils to help relieve congestion and promote easier breathing.

7. **Nasal Irrigation**:
   - Use saline nasal irrigation or saline nasal sprays to help clear nasal passages and relieve congestion.

8. **Humidification**:
   - Use a humidifier in your home to add moisture to the air and prevent dryness, which can exacerbate respiratory symptoms.

9. **Pain Relief**:
   - Use over-the-counter pain relievers such as acetaminophen or ibuprofen to reduce fever and alleviate aches and pains if needed.

10. **Limit Exposure**:
    - Avoid close contact with sick individuals and practice good hygiene habits such as frequent handwashing to prevent the spread of cold and flu viruses.

11. **Manage Stress**:
   - Practice stress-reducing techniques such as deep breathing, meditation, yoga, or gentle exercise to help manage stress and support immune function.

12. **Monitor Symptoms**:
   - Keep track of your symptoms and seek medical attention if they worsen or if you have concerns about your health.

By incorporating these self-care practices into your routine, you can empower yourself to effectively manage cold and flu symptoms, support your immune system, and promote overall well-being. However, if your symptoms persist or worsen, it's important to consult with a healthcare professional for proper evaluation and treatment.

www.ingramcontent.com/pod-product-compliance
Lightning Source LLC
Chambersburg PA
CBHW050304230526
45471CB00005B/2017